THE *Skinny* SLOW COOKER SOUP RECIPE BOOK

Simple, Healthy & Delicious Low Calorie Soup Recipes For Your Slow Cooker. All Under 100, 200 & 300 Calories.

CookNation

The Skinny Slow Cooker Soup Recipe Book
Simple, Healthy & Delicious Low Calorie Soup
Recipes For Your Slow Cooker. All Under 100, 200
& 300 Calories.

A Bell & Mackenzie Publication
First published in 2014 by Bell & Mackenzie Publishing
Limited.
Copyright © Bell & Mackenzie Publishing 2014

ISBN 978-1-909-855-30-4

A CIP catalogue record of this book is available from the
British Library

Disclaimer
The information and advice in this book is intended as
a guide only. If using the recipes as part of a diet, any
individual should independently seek the advice of a
doctor or health professional before embarking on any
diet or weight loss plan. We do not recommend a calorie
controlled diet if you are pregnant, breastfeeding, elderly
or under 18 years of age. Some recipes may contain nuts or
traces of nuts. Those suffering from any allergies associated
with nuts should avoid any recipes containing nuts or nut
based oils.

Contents

Contents

Contents

Introduction

Slow cookers are one of the most versatile appliances in the kitchen. They allow us to cook nearly everything from roasts and stews to side dishes and desserts but perhaps one of the most rewarding, healthy and simplest of dishes that the slow cooker can create is soup.

Soup can come in many guises – a traditional warming broth, a light and simple minestrone or a creamy chicken laksa. The list of recipes and options are endless and the slow cooker is the perfect vessel to create your dish whatever the time of year. The slow cooker uses moist heat to create full flavour, all in one pot, allowing you to get on with what's important.

The Skinny Slow Cooker Soup recipes focus on healthy fresh ingredients, are low in calories, simple to prepare and full of flavour. Our skinny soups are perfect as part of a balanced diet and can be instrumental in helping you lose weight or maintain your figure without compromising on flavour, taste or leaving you feeling hungry. All our recipes fall under either 100, 200 or 300 calories per serving which makes them the perfect partner to any calorie controlled diet.

Making soup in a slow cooker is incredibly easy. Preparation time for all our recipes is less than 15 minutes. You can also make use of whatever leftovers you have in the kitchen and nearly all our soups can be frozen and stored for another time.

If you are looking for some new ideas for soup making to help you lose weight, control your diet or to serve up a healthy balanced dish for your family then you will find inspiration here.

We hope you enjoy this collection of skinny slow cooker soups.

What Is A Skinny Soup?
Simply put a 'skinny' soup is one of our delicious slow cooker soup recipes each falling below either 100, 200 or 300 calories per serving. By calculating the number of calories for each dish we've made it easy for you to count your daily calorie intake as part of a controlled diet or a balanced healthy eating plan.

Preparation
All the recipes should take no longer than 10-15 minutes to prepare. Browning some of the vegetables and/or meat will make a difference to the taste of your recipe, but if you really don't have the time, don't worry - it will still taste great.

All meat and vegetables should be cut into even sized pieces unless stated in the recipes. Some ingredients can take longer to cook than others, particularly root vegetables, but that has been allowed for in the cooking time.

As much as possible, meat should be trimmed of visible fat and the skin removed.

Slow Cooker Tips
• All cooking times are a guide. Make sure you get to know your own slow cooker so that you can adjust timings accordingly.
• Read the manufacturers operating instructions as appliances can vary. For example, some recommend preheating the slow cooker for 20 minutes before use whilst others advocate switching on only when you are ready to start cooking.
• A spray of low calorie cooking oil in the cooker before adding ingredients will help with cleaning or you can buy liners.
• Don't be tempted to regularly lift the lid of your appliance while cooking. The seal that is made with the lid on is all part of the slow cooking process.

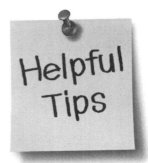

Each time you do lift the lid you may need to increase the cooking time.
• Removing the lid at the end of the cooking time can be useful to thicken up a soup by adding additional cooking time and continuing to cook without the lid on. On the other hand if the soup is too thick removing the lid and adding a little more liquid can help.
• Where possible always add hot liquids to your slow cooker, not cold.
• Do not overfill your slow cooker.
• Allow the inner dish of your slow cooker to completely cool before cleaning. Any stubborn marks can usually be removed after a period of soaking in hot soapy water.
• Be confident with your cooking. Feel free to use substitutes to suit your own taste and don't let a missing

herb or spice stop you making a meal - you'll almost always be able to find something to replace it.

Our Recipes
The recipes in this book are all low calorie soups serving 4, which makes it easier for you to monitor your overall daily calorie intake as well as those you are cooking for. The recommended daily calories are approximately 2000 for women and 2500 for men.

Broadly speaking, by consuming the recommended levels of calories each day you should maintain your current weight. Reducing the number of calories (a calorie deficit) will result in losing weight. This happens because the body begins to use fat stores for energy to make up the reduction in calories, which in turn results in weight loss. We have already counted the calories for each dish making it easy for you to fit this into your daily eating plan whether you want to lose weight, maintain your current figure or are just looking for some great-tasting, skinny slow cooker soups.

I'm Already On A Diet. Can I Use These Recipes?
Yes of course. All the recipes can be great accompaniments to many of the popular calorie-counting diets. We all know that sometimes dieting can result in hunger pangs, cravings and boredom from eating the same old foods day in and day out. Skinny slow cooker soups can break that cycle by providing healthy and interesting soups, which will satisfy you for hours afterwards.

I Am Only Cooking For One. Will This Book Work For Me?
Yes. To make the best use of each dish we have made

all servings for four people. Remember you can always refrigerate or freeze portions for another day if you are just cooking for one.

Soup Is Just For Cold Winter Nights, Right?

Wrong! While there is nothing better than a bowl of comforting steaming hot broth on a miserable winter's day, soup isn't just for dark cold nights. It can be a vibrant and refreshing alternative on the brightest and hottest of days, and makes use of the best seasonal ingredients all year round.

What Makes A Great Soup?

Thankfully you don't have to be a great chef to make an incredible soup in your slow cooker. There are however a few key elements to making a great soup.

• **The Base:** the start to most soups requires a few vegetables to give your soup a rounded flavour. Onions, carrots and celery are a great start.

• **Ingredients:** Soup is so versatile that almost any ingredient can be used whether you are looking for a meaty protein packed dish, an Asian seafood soup, or a thick vegetarian broth using beans and pulses. Certain ingredients will change the consistency of your soup too, for example potatoes and lentils will thicken, while adding some single cream or milk will make it smoother.

• **Seasoning:** Most soups will require some seasoning. Be careful when choosing your stock that it is not overly high in its sodium content. There are also many popular herbs that compliment soups such as marjoram, thyme, parsley, sage, rosemary, oregano and of course salt and pepper. You should also feel free to experiment. For example: Garlic, ginger and coriander can work well in Asian soups while cumin, turmeric or garam masala can give an authentic Indian feel to your dish.

Garnish: There is nothing better than serving a homemade soup with a little garnish, which not only looks the part but also adds an extra taste. Depending on your dish, freshly chopped herbs, croutons, fat free Greek yoghurt, low fat crème fraiche or freshly grated Parmesan are all great finishing touches.

All Recipes Are A Guide Only
All the recipes in this book are a guide only. You may need to alter quantities and cooking times to suit your own appliance – do not overfill your slow cooker.

Consistency is also a question of personal preference. Some recipes suggest the best consistency to use; others leave it to your own personal taste. Feel free to experiment by adding more or less liquid to suit your own taste.

STOCK

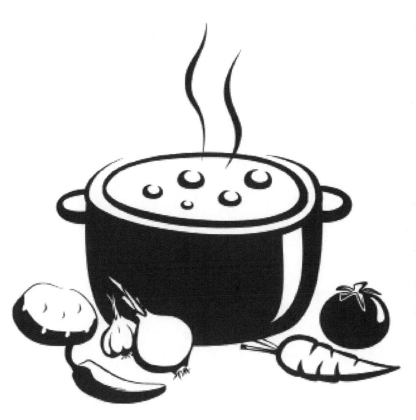

Homemade stock is not essential for any soup making, but you will find it can add additional depth of taste and further improve the flavour of some dishes. Having said that, shop bought stock has vastly improved in recent times and you may well decide making your own stock isn't worth the time for the comparable result. If you do use shop bought stock (which most people do) avoid buying budget options and anything too high in sodium.

For those of you who want to make stock from scratch, to follow are a few simple stock recipes to start with which you can quickly make on the stove-top.

Basic Vegetable Stock

Serves 4

Method:

- Gently sauté the onions, leeks, carrots and fennel in the olive oil for a few minutes in a large lidded saucepan.
- Add all the other ingredients, cover and bring to the boil. Leave to gently simmer for 20 minutes with the lid on.
- Allow to cool for a little while.
- Pour the contents through a sieve and store the finished stock liquid in the fridge for a couple of days or freeze in batches.

Ingredients:

1 tbsp olive oil
1 onion, chopped
1 leek, chopped
1 carrot, chopped
1 small bulb fennel, chopped
3 garlic cloves, crushed
1 tbsp black peppercorns
75g/3oz mushrooms
2 sticks celery, chopped
3 tomatoes, diced
2 tbsp freshly chopped flat leaf parsley
2 bay leaves
3lt/12 cups water

Basic Chicken Stock
Serves 4

Ingredients:

1 tbsp olive oil
1 left over roast chicken carcass
2 carrots, chopped
2 onions, halved
2 stalks celery, chopped
10 black peppercorns
2 bay leaves
2 tbsp freshly chopped parsley
1 tsp freshly chopped thyme
3lt/12 cups water

Method:

• Gently sauté the onions, leeks, carrots and fennel in the olive oil for a few minutes in a large lidded saucepan.
• Add all the other ingredients, cover and bring to the boil. Leave to gently simmer for 20 minutes with the lid on.
• Allow to cool for a little while.
• Pour the contents through a sieve and store the finished stock liquid in the fridge for a couple of days or freeze in batches.

Basic Fish Stock
Serves 4

Method:

- Gently sauté the carrots, leeks and fennel in the olive oil for a few minutes in a large lidded saucepan.
- Clean the fish bones to ensure there is no blood as this can 'spoil' the stock.
- Add all the other ingredients, cover and bring to the boil. Leave to very gently simmer for 1hr with the lid on.
- Allow to cool for a little while.
- Pour the contents through a sieve and store the finished stock liquid in the fridge for a couple of days or freeze in batches.
- You may find you need to skim a little fat from the top of the stock after cooking.

Ingredients:

1 tbsp olive oil
450g/1lb fish bones, heads carcasses etc (avoid oily fish when making stock)
4 leeks, chopped
1 fennel bulb, chopped
4 carrots, chopped
2 tbsp freshly chopped parsley
250ml/1 cup dry white wine
2.5lt/10 cups water

VEGETABLE
SOUPS

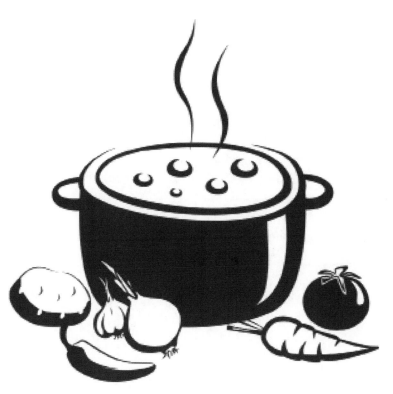

The Skinny **SLOW**
COOKER
SOUP
RECIPE BOOK

Chickpea & Tomato Soup
Serves 4

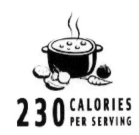

230 CALORIES PER SERVING

Ingredients:

2 leeks, chopped
2 garlic cloves, crushed
125g/4oz courgettes/
zucchini sliced
400g/14oz tinned
chickpeas, drained
400g/14oz tinned chopped
tomatoes
2 tbsp tomato puree/paste
500ml/2 cups vegetable
stock/broth
125g/4oz tenderstem
broccoli, roughly chopped
Salt & pepper to taste
Low cal cooking oil spray

Method:

• Preheat the slow cooker while you prepare the ingredients.
• Gently sauté the leeks & garlic in a little low cal oil for a few minutes until the leeks soften.
• Add all the ingredients to the slow cooker. Combine well, cover and leave to cook on high for 1-1½ hours or until the vegetables are cooked through.
• Check the seasoning and serve.

Also known as garbanzo beans, chickpeas are a good source of protein.

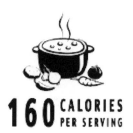

Beetroot Soup
Serves 4

160 CALORIES PER SERVING

Method:

- Preheat the slow cooker while you prepare the ingredients.
- Gently sauté the onion & cumin seeds in a little low cal oil for a few minutes until the onions soften.
- Add all the ingredients to the slow cooker, except the Greek yoghurt. Combine well, cover and leave to cook on high for 1-1½ hours or until the vegetables are cooked through.
- Blend to a smooth consistency.
- Check the seasoning and serve with a dollop of yoghurt in the middle of each bowl.

Ingredients:

1 onion, chopped
1 tsp cumin seeds
150g/5oz potatoes, chopped
400g/14oz beetroot, cubed
750ml/3 cups vegetable stock/broth
1 tsp dried basil or oregano
1 tsp lemon juice
4 tbsp fat free Greek yoghurt
Salt & pepper to taste
Low cal cooking oil spray

This soup has a fantastic vibrant colour, which is contrasted by a generous dollop of white yoghurt.

Savoury Apple & Apricot Soup
Serves 4

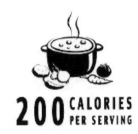

200 CALORIES PER SERVING

Ingredients:

1 onion, chopped
125g/4oz dried apricots, chopped
500g/1lb 2oz eating apples, peeled, cored & finely chopped
750ml/3 cups vegetable stock/broth
½ tsp nutmeg
1 tbsp lemon juice
4 tbsp fat free Greek yoghurt
Salt & pepper to taste
Low cal cooking oil spray

Method:

• Preheat the slow cooker while you prepare the ingredients.
• Gently sauté the onions in a little low cal oil for a few minutes until softened.
• Add all the ingredients to the slow cooker, except the Greek yoghurt. Combine well, cover and leave to cook on high for 1-1½ hours or until the vegetables and apples are cooked through.
• Blend to a smooth consistency.
• Check the seasoning and serve with a dollop of yoghurt in the middle of each bowl.

You could also add a pinch of ground ginger and/or cinnamon to this soup if you have it to hand.

Three Bean Soup

Serves 4

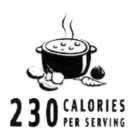

230 CALORIES PER SERVING

Method:

- Preheat the slow cooker while you prepare the ingredients.
- Gently sauté the leeks, onion & garlic in a little low cal oil for a few minutes until softened.
- Add all the ingredients to the slow cooker. Combine well, cover and leave to cook on high for 1-1½ hours or until the vegetables are cooked through.
- Check the seasoning and serve.

Ingredients:

2 leeks, sliced
1 onion, sliced
2 garlic cloves, crushed
1 carrot, chopped
1 green chilli, finely chopped
400g/14oz tinned mixed beans, drained
125g/4oz courgettes/ zucchini sliced
2 tbsp tomato puree/paste
1lt/4 cups vegetable stock/ broth
Salt & pepper to taste
Low cal cooking oil spray

If you don't have fresh chillies, use a little chilli powder or cayenne pepper.

Simple Lentil Soup
Serves 4

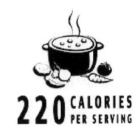

220 CALORIES PER SERVING

Ingredients:

1 onion, chopped
2 celery sticks, chopped
2 garlic cloves, crushed
1 carrot, chopped
225g/8oz red lentils
1 bay leaf
1lt/4 cups vegetable stock/broth
4 tsp low fat crème fraiche
Salt & pepper to taste
Low cal cooking oil spray

Method:

• Preheat the slow cooker while you prepare the ingredients.
• Gently sauté the onion, celery & garlic in a little low cal oil for a few minutes until the onions soften.
• Add all the ingredients to the slow cooker, except the crème fraiche. Combine well, cover and leave to cook on high for 1-2 hours or until the vegetables are cooked through and the lentils are tender.
• Remove the bay leaf and blend the soup to a smooth consistency.
• Check the seasoning and serve with a tsp of crème fraiche in the middle of each bowl.

You could garnish with freshly chopped coriander/cilantro or flat leaf parsley if you have it to hand.

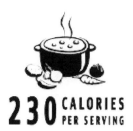

Split Pea Soup
Serves 4

230 CALORIES PER SERVING

Method:

- Preheat the slow cooker while you prepare the ingredients.
- Gently sauté the onion, celery & garlic in a little low cal oil for a few minutes until the onions soften.
- Add all the ingredients to the slow cooker. Combine well, cover and leave to cook on high for 1-2 hours or until the vegetables are cooked through and the split peas are tender.
- Blend the soup to a smooth consistency, season and serve.

Ingredients:

2 onions, chopped
2 celery sticks, chopped
2 garlic cloves, crushed
2 carrots, chopped
1 turnip, chopped
225g/8oz pre-soaked yellow split peas
2 tsp mixed dried herbs
1lt/4 cups vegetable stock/ broth
Salt & pepper to taste
Low cal cooking oil spray

Thyme, basil or oregano will all work in this soup if you don't have dried mixed herbs.

25

Pea & Mint Soup
Serves 4

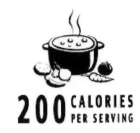

200 CALORIES
PER SERVING

Ingredients:

2 onions, chopped
2 garlic cloves, crushed
200g/7oz potatoes,
chopped
1 tsp medium curry
powder
500g/1lb 2oz peas
3 tbsp freshly chopped
mint
750ml/3 cups vegetable
stock/broth
250ml/1 cup semi
skimmed/half fat milk
Salt & pepper to taste
Low cal cooking oil spray

Method:

• Preheat the slow cooker while you prepare the ingredients.
• Gently sauté the onion & garlic in a little low cal oil for a few minutes until the onions soften.
• Add all the ingredients to the slow cooker. Combine well, cover and leave to cook on high for 1-1½ hours or until the vegetables are tender.
• Blend the soup to a smooth consistency, season and serve.

Reserve a little of the chopped mint as a garnish.

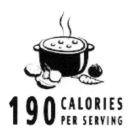

Sweet Potato & Orange Soup

Serves 4

190 CALORIES PER SERVING

Method:

- Preheat the slow cooker while you prepare the ingredients.
- Gently sauté the onion in a little low cal oil for a few minutes until softened.
- Add all the ingredients to the slow cooker. Combine well, cover and leave to cook on high for 1-1½ hours or until the vegetables are tender.
- Blend the soup to a smooth consistency, season and serve.

Ingredients:

2 onions, chopped
2 carrots, chopped
500g/1lb 2oz sweet potatoes, chopped
750ml/3 cups vegetable stock/broth
250ml/1 cup fresh orange juice
Salt & pepper to taste
Low cal cooking oil spray

Freshly chopped coriander/ cilantro makes a really worthwhile addition to this soup.

27

Lentil & Ginger Chowder

Serves 4

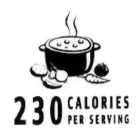

230 CALORIES PER SERVING

Ingredients:

1 onion, chopped
2 garlic cloves, crushed
1 tbsp freshly grated ginger
1 tbsp soy sauce
200g/7oz sweetcorn
2 celery sticks
225g/8oz red lentils
1lt/4 cups vegetable stock/broth
2 red chillies, finely chopped
Salt & pepper to taste
Low cal cooking oil spray

Method:

• Preheat the slow cooker while you prepare the ingredients.
• Gently sauté the onion & garlic in a little low cal oil for a few minutes until the onions soften.
• Add all the ingredients to the slow cooker, except the chopped chilli. Combine well, cover and leave to cook on high for 1-2 hours or until the vegetables are cooked through and the lentils are tender.
• Remove 2 ladles of soup and use a blender to blend this to a smooth consistency. Return the blended portion to the rest of the soup.
• Check the seasoning and serve with the red chilli sprinkled over the top as a garnish.

Two red chillies will give this soup quite a 'kick'. You may want to alter the quantity to suit your own taste!

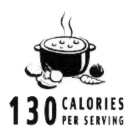

Honey & Carrot Soup
Serves 4

130 CALORIES PER SERVING

Method:

- Preheat the slow cooker while you prepare the ingredients.
- Gently sauté the onions in a little low cal oil for a few minutes until softened.
- Add all the ingredients to the slow cooker. Combine well, cover and leave to cook on high for 1-1½ hours or until the vegetables are tender.
- Blend the soup to a smooth consistency, season and serve.

Ingredients:

1 onion, chopped
500g/1lb 2oz carrots, chopped
125g/4oz potatoes, chopped
1lt/4 cups vegetable stock/ broth
1 tsp runny honey
Salt & pepper to taste
Low cal cooking oil spray

Freshly chopped chives and/or a swirl of single cream make a lovely garnish to this soup.

Carrot & Cumin Seed Soup
Serves 4

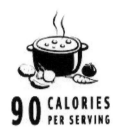

90 CALORIES PER SERVING

Ingredients:

1 onion, chopped
½ tsp cumin seeds
1 garlic clove, crushed
400g/14oz carrots, chopped
125g/4oz potatoes, chopped
1 parsnip, chopped
750ml/3 cups vegetable stock/broth
250ml/1 cup semi skimmed/half fat milk
2 tsp tomato puree/paste
Salt & pepper to taste
Low cal cooking oil spray

Method:

• Preheat the slow cooker while you prepare the ingredients.
• Gently sauté the onions, cumin seeds & garlic in a little low cal oil for a few minutes until softened.
• Add all the ingredients to the slow cooker. Combine well, cover and leave to cook on high for 1-1½ hours or until the vegetables are tender.
• Blend the soup to a smooth consistency, season and serve.

Ground cumin also works equally well in this recipe.

Apple & Celery Soup

Serves 4

140 CALORIES PER SERVING

Method:

- Preheat the slow cooker while you prepare the ingredients.
- Gently sauté the onion & celery in a little low cal oil for a few minutes until softened.
- Add all the ingredients to the slow cooker, except the lemon wedges. Combine well, cover and leave to cook on high for 1-1½ hours or until the vegetables and apples are tender.
- Blend the soup to a smooth consistency, season and serve with the lemon wedges.

Ingredients:

1 onion, chopped
4 sticks celery, chopped
300g/11oz eating apples, peeled, cored & chopped
300g/11oz carrots, chopped
1lt/4 cups vegetable stock/broth
1 tsp each brown sugar
½ tsp salt
2 tbsp tomato puree/paste
Lemon wedges to serve
Salt & pepper to taste
Low cal cooking oil spray

This is a really light, fresh-tasting soup.

Curried Potato Soup
Serves 4

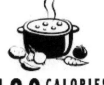

180 CALORIES PER SERVING

Ingredients:

1 onion, chopped
2 garlic cloves, crushed
1 tbsp medium curry powder
400g/14oz potatoes, peeled & cut into chunks
200g/7oz peas
1lt/4 cups vegetable stock/ broth
3 tbsp fat free Greek yoghurt
Lemon wedges to serve
Salt & pepper to taste
Low cal cooking oil spray

Method:

• Preheat the slow cooker while you prepare the ingredients.
• Gently sauté the onion & garlic in a little low cal oil for a few minutes until softened.
• Add all the ingredients to the slow cooker, except the Greek yoghurt. Combine well, cover and leave to cook on high for 1-1½ hours or until the potatoes are tender but not completely falling apart.
• Remove 2 ladles of soup and use a blender to blend this to a smooth consistency. Return the blended portion to the rest of the soup.
• Stir through the yoghurt, combine well, season and serve.

Finely chopped red chillies make a good garnish for this soup if you want to add additional 'heat'.

Vegetable Daal Soup

Serves 4

175 CALORIES PER SERVING

Method:

• Preheat the slow cooker while you prepare the ingredients.

• Gently sauté the onion & garlic in a little low cal oil for a few minutes until softened.

• Add all the ingredients to the slow cooker. Combine well, cover and leave to cook on high for 1-2 hours or until the lentils and vegetables are tender.

• Blend to a smooth consistency, season and serve.

Ingredients:

1 onion, chopped
2 garlic cloves, crushed
1 tbsp medium curry powder
200g/7oz tinned chopped tomatoes
200g/7oz potatoes, chopped
200g/7oz carrots, chopped
125g/4oz red lentils
750ml/3 cups vegetable stock/broth
Salt & pepper to taste
Low cal cooking oil spray

A swirl of milk and chopped chives make a good garnish for this soup too.

33

Easy Cauliflower Cheese Soup
Serves 4

190 CALORIES PER SERVING

Ingredients:

1 onion, chopped
1 large cauliflower, broken into florets
125g/4oz potatoes, chopped
750ml/3 cups vegetable stock/broth
250ml/1 cup semi skimmed/halt fat milk
125g/4oz low fat cheddar cheese, grated
Salt & pepper to taste
Low cal cooking oil spray

Method:

• Preheat the slow cooker while you prepare the ingredients.
• Gently sauté the onion in a little low cal oil for a few minutes until softened.
• Add all the ingredients to the slow cooker, except the grated cheese. Combine well, cover and leave to cook on high for 1-1½ hours or until the vegetables are tender.
• Blend to a smooth consistency and sprinkle the grated cheese evenly into each bowl.
• Season and serve.

Chopped flat leaf parsley adds a nice garnish to this soup.

34

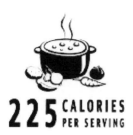

Sundried Tomato & Bean Soup

Serves 4

225 CALORIES PER SERVING

Method:

- Preheat the slow cooker while you prepare the ingredients.
- Gently sauté the onion & garlic in a little low cal oil for a few minutes until softened.
- Add all the ingredients to the slow cooker. Combine well, cover and leave to cook on high for 1-1½ hours or until the potatoes are tender.
- Remove 2 ladles of soup and use a blender to blend this to a smooth consistency. Return the blended portion to the rest of the soup.
- Combine well, season and serve.

Ingredients:

2 onions, chopped
2 garlic cloves, crushed
400g/14oz borlotti beans, drained
150g/5oz potatoes, chopped
4 tbsp sundried tomato puree/paste
1lt/4 cups vegetable stock/broth
Salt & pepper to taste
Low cal cooking oil spray

Use any type of bean you prefer for this soup. Cannellini or Butter beans will work just as well.

Pea, Leek & Garlic Soup
Serves 4

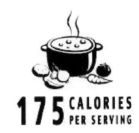

175 CALORIES PER SERVING

Ingredients:

2 leeks, chopped
4 garlic cloves, crushed
400g/14oz peas
125g/4oz potatoes, chopped
1lt/4 cups vegetable stock/broth
Salt & pepper to taste
Low cal cooking oil spray

Method:

• Preheat the slow cooker while you prepare the ingredients.
• Gently sauté the leeks & garlic in a little low cal oil for a few minutes until the leeks soften.
• Add all the ingredients to the slow cooker. Combine well, cover and leave to cook on high for 1-1½ hours or until the vegetables are tender.
• Blend the soup to a smooth consistency, season and serve.

Freshly chopped mint makes a lovely garnish to this soup.

Watercress & Blue Cheese Soup

Serves 4

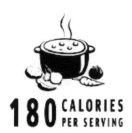

180 CALORIES
PER SERVING

Method:

- Preheat the slow cooker while you prepare the ingredients.
- Add all the ingredients to the slow cooker, except the cheese. Combine well, cover and leave to cook on high for 1-1½ hours or until the potatoes are tender.
- Crumble the cheese into the soup and blend to a smooth consistency.
- Season and serve with a few sprigs of watercress on top.

Ingredients:

300g/12oz watercress
125g/4oz potatoes, chopped
750ml/3 cups vegetable stock/broth
250ml/1 cup semi skimmed/half fat milk
125g/4oz blue cheese, crumbled
Salt & pepper to taste
Low cal cooking oil spray

Use whichever type of blue cheese you prefer. Stilton is a national favourite.

Celeriac Soup
Serves 4

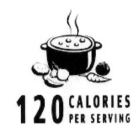

120 CALORIES PER SERVING

Ingredients:

1 onion, chopped
½ tsp fennel seeds
1 garlic clove, crushed
500g/1lb 2oz celeriac,
chopped
1lt/4 cups vegetable stock/
broth
4 tsp low fat crème fraiche
Salt & pepper to taste
Low cal cooking oil spray

Method:

- Preheat the slow cooker while you prepare the ingredients.
- Gently sauté the onion, fennel seeds & garlic in a little low cal oil for a few minutes until the onions soften.
- Add all the ingredients to the slow cooker, except the crème fraiche. Combine well, cover and leave to cook on high for 1-1½ hours or until the celeriac is tender.
- Blend the soup to a smooth consistency, season and serve with a teaspoon of crème fraiche in the centre of each bowl.

Plenty of black pepper when serving complements this soup.

38

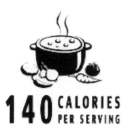

Creamy Mushroom Soup
Serves 4

140 CALORIES PER SERVING

Method:

- Preheat the slow cooker while you prepare the ingredients.
- Gently sauté the onions in a little low cal oil for a few minutes until softened.
- Add all the ingredients to the slow cooker, except the crème fraiche. Combine well, cover and leave to cook on high for 1-1½ hours or until the potatoes are tender.
- Blend the soup to a smooth consistency.
- Season and serve with a teaspoon of crème fraiche stirred through each bowl.

Ingredients:

1 onion, chopped
½ tsp nutmeg
125g/4oz potatoes, chopped
500g/1lb 2oz mushrooms, sliced
750ml/3 cups vegetable stock/broth
250ml/1 cup semi skimmed/half fat milk
4 tsp low fat crème fraiche
Salt & pepper to taste
Low cal cooking oil spray

Freshly chopped tarragon or chives make a good garnish for this soup.

Onion & Squash Soup
Serves 4

150 CALORIES PER SERVING

Ingredients:

2 onions, chopped
2 garlic cloves, crushed
1 carrot, chopped
1 carrot, finely grated
**500g/1lb 2oz butternut
squash flesh, diced**
**1lt/4 cups vegetable stock/
broth**
Salt & pepper to taste
Low cal cooking oil spray

Method:

- Preheat the slow cooker while you prepare the ingredients.
- Gently sauté the onion & garlic in a little low cal oil for a few minutes until the onions soften.
- Add all the ingredients to the slow cooker, except the grated carrot. Combine well, cover and leave to cook on high for 1-1½ hours or until the vegetables are tender.
- Blend the soup to a smooth consistency.
- Season and serve with the grated carrot on top.

Freshly chopped chives make a good garnish for this soup.

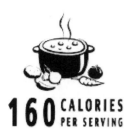

Pumpkin & Nutmeg Soup
Serves 4

160 CALORIES PER SERVING

Method:

- Preheat the slow cooker while you prepare the ingredients.
- Gently sauté the onion & garlic in a little low cal oil for a few minutes until softened.
- Add all the ingredients to the slow cooker. Combine well, cover and leave to cook on high for 1-1½ hours or until the pumpkin is tender.
- Blend the soup to a smooth consistency, season and serve.

Ingredients:

1 onion, chopped
1 garlic clove, crushed
500g/1lb 2oz pumpkin flesh, diced
½ tsp nutmeg
500ml/2 cups semi skimmed/half fat milk
500ml/ 2 cups vegetable stock/broth
Salt & pepper to taste
Low cal cooking oil spray

A pinch of cinnamon complements this soup really well too.

Potato & Parsnip Soup
Serves 4

175 CALORIES PER SERVING

Ingredients:

1 onion, chopped
1 garlic clove, crushed
400g/14oz potatoes, diced
200g/7oz parsnip,
chopped
1 tsp mixed herbs
1lt/4 cups vegetable stock/
broth
Salt & pepper to taste
Low cal cooking oil spray

Method:

• Preheat the slow cooker while you prepare the ingredients.
• Gently sauté the onion & garlic in a little low cal oil for a few minutes until the onions soften.
• Add all the ingredients to the slow cooker. Combine well, cover and leave to cook on high for 1-1½ hours or until the potatoes and parsnips are tender.
• Blend the soup to a smooth consistency, season and serve.

Serve with chopped flat leaf parsley if you have any to hand.

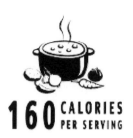

Celeriac & Spinach Soup

Serves 4

160 CALORIES PER SERVING

Method:

- Preheat the slow cooker while you prepare the ingredients.
- First quickly toast the pine nuts in a dry pan for a minute or two, shaking continuously until they turn golden brown.
- Remove the pine nuts from the pan and chop.
- Use the same pan to gently sauté the onion & garlic in a little low cal oil for a few minutes until the onions soften.
- Add all the ingredients to the slow cooker, except the pine nuts. Combine well, cover and leave to cook on high for 1-1½ hours or until the celeriac is tender.
- Blend the soup to a smooth consistency, season and serve with the pine nuts sprinkled on top.

You could use chopped toasted pumpkin seeds rather than pine nuts if you prefer for the garnish.

Ingredients:

2 tbsp pine nuts
1 onion, chopped
1 garlic clove, crushed
500g/1lb 2oz celeriac, chopped
200g/7oz spinach leaves, roughly chopped
750ml/3 cups vegetable stock/broth
250ml/1 cup semi skimmed/half fat milk
Salt & pepper to taste
Low cal cooking oil spray

Spinach & Cabbage Soup
Serves 4

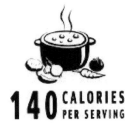

140 CALORIES PER SERVING

Ingredients:

1 leek, chopped
1 onion, chopped
2 garlic cloves, crushed
200g/7oz spinach, roughly chopped
1 green pointed cabbage, chopped
125g/4oz rice
1lt/4 cups vegetable stock/broth
Salt & pepper to taste
Low cal cooking oil spray

Method:

• Preheat the slow cooker while you prepare the ingredients.
• Gently sauté the leeks, onions & garlic in a little low cal oil for a few minutes until softened.
• Add all the ingredients to the slow cooker. Combine well, cover and leave to cook on high for 1-1½ hours or until the vegetables and rice are tender.
• Blend the soup to a smooth consistency, season and serve.

You can use any other kind of cabbage you have to hand, but firm pointed cabbage is particularly good.

44

Classic Vegetable Soup

Serves 4

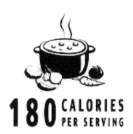

180 CALORIES PER SERVING

Method:

- Preheat the slow cooker while you prepare the ingredients.
- Gently sauté the leek, onion & garlic in a little low cal oil for a few minutes until softened.
- Add all the ingredients to the slow cooker. Combine well, cover and leave to cook on high for 1-1½ hours or until the vegetables are tender.
- Blend the soup to a smooth consistency, season and serve.

Ingredients:

1 leek, chopped
1 onion, chopped
2 garlic cloves, crushed
200g/7oz carrots, chopped
200g/7oz parsnip, chopped
200g/7oz potatoes, chopped
1lt/4 cups vegetable stock/ broth
Salt & pepper to taste
Low cal cooking oil spray

This is a classic smooth vegetable soup. You could leave it chunky if you prefer.

Garlic Root Soup
Serves 4

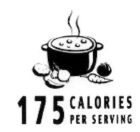

175 CALORIES PER SERVING

Ingredients:

1 onion, chopped
8 garlic cloves, crushed
200g/7oz sweet potatoes, chopped
200g/7oz parsnip, chopped
200g/7oz potatoes, chopped
1lt/4 cups vegetable stock/ broth
Salt & pepper to taste
Low cal cooking oil spray

Method:

• Preheat the slow cooker while you prepare the ingredients.
• Gently sauté the onions & garlic in a little low cal oil for a few minutes until softened.
• Add all the ingredients to the slow cooker. Combine well, cover and leave to cook on high for 1-1½ hours or until the vegetables are tender.
• Blend the soup to a smooth consistency, season and serve.

For a different twist use squash rather than sweet potatoes.

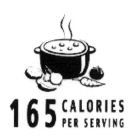

Tomato Soup
Serves 4

165 CALORIES PER SERVING

Method:

- Preheat the slow cooker while you prepare the ingredients.
- Gently sauté the onion & garlic in a little low cal oil for a few minutes until the onions soften.
- Add all the ingredients to the slow cooker. Combine well, cover and leave to cook on high for 1-1½ hours or until the vegetables are tender.
- Blend the soup to a smooth consistency, season and serve.

Ingredients:

1 onion, chopped
2 garlic cloves, crushed
200g/7oz potatoes, chopped
200g/7oz fresh ripe tomatoes, chopped
400g/14oz tinned chopped tomatoes
1 tsp dried basil
½ tsp salt
1 tsp brown sugar
250ml/1 cup vegetable stock/broth
Salt & pepper to taste
Low cal cooking oil spray

The salt and sugar will help balance the acidity of the tomatoes. Use a little more if needed.

47

Russian Borscht

Serves 4

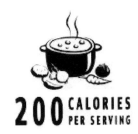

200 CALORIES PER SERVING

Ingredients:

1 onion, chopped
1 stick celery, chopped
1 carrot, chopped
400g/14oz tinned chopped tomatoes
500ml/2 cup vegetable stock/broth
2 bay leaves
200g/7oz cooked beetroot, grated
4 tbsp fat free Greek yoghurt
Salt & pepper to taste
Low cal cooking oil spray

Method:

• Preheat the slow cooker while you prepare the ingredients.
• Gently sauté the onion & celery in a little low cal oil for a few minutes until the onions soften.
• Add all the ingredients to the slow cooker, except the beetroot & Greek yoghurt. Combine well, cover and leave to cook on high for 1-1½ hours or until the vegetables are tender.
• Remove the bay leaves, blend the soup to a smooth consistency and return to the slow cooker.
• Add the grated beetroot and warm through for 20-30 minutes.
• Season and serve with a dollop of Greek yoghurt in the middle of each bowl.

You could add lemon wedges to this soup when you serve.

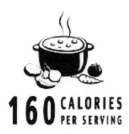

Porcini Soup
Serves 4

160 CALORIES PER SERVING

Method:

- Preheat the slow cooker while you prepare the ingredients.
- Gently sauté the onion & garlic in a little low cal oil for a few minutes until the onions soften.
- Add all the ingredients to the slow cooker. Combine well, cover and leave to cook on high for 1-1½ hours or until the potatoes are tender.
- Blend the soup to a smooth consistency, season and serve.

Ingredients:

1 onion, chopped
2 garlic cloves, crushed
75g/3oz dried porcini mushrooms, chopped
125g/4oz potatoes, chopped
300g/11oz mushrooms, sliced
750ml/3 cups vegetable stock/broth
250ml/1 cup semi skimmed/half fat milk
Salt & pepper to taste
Low cal cooking oil spray

You could add two teaspoons of chopped rosemary to this soup either as an ingredient or as a serving garnish.

Simple Minestrone Soup
Serves 4

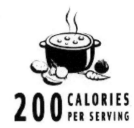

200 CALORIES PER SERVING

Ingredients:

1 onion, chopped
2 celery sticks, finely chopped
2 carrots, finely chopped
400g/14oz tinned chopped tomatoes
75g/3oz dried spaghetti, roughly broken up
1lt/4 cups vegetable stock/broth
2 tbsp freshly grated Parmesan cheese
Salt & pepper to taste
Low cal cooking oil spray

Method:

• Preheat the slow cooker while you prepare the ingredients.
• Gently sauté the onion & celery in a little low cal oil for a few minutes until the onions soften.
• Add all the ingredients to the slow cooker, except the grated Parmesan cheese. Combine well, cover and leave to cook on high for 1-1½ hours or until the vegetables & pasta are tender.
• Season and serve with Parmesan sprinkled over the top.

Any type of small pasta shapes will work fine for this simple minestrone style soup.

Courgette Soup

Serves 4

90 CALORIES PER SERVING

Method:

- Preheat the slow cooker while you prepare the ingredients.
- Gently sauté the onion & garlic in a little low cal oil for a few minutes until the onions soften.
- Add all the ingredients to the slow cooker. Combine well, cover and leave to cook on high for 1-1½ hours or until the vegetables are tender.
- Blend the soup to a smooth consistency, season and serve.

Ingredients:

1 onion, chopped
2 garlic cloves, crushed
400g/14oz courgettes, sliced
1 tsp dried oregano or basil
750ml/3 cups vegetable stock/broth
250ml/1 cup semi skimmed/half fat milk
Salt & pepper to taste
Low cal cooking oil spray

A swirl of cream and/or some fresh basil are great with this soup.

POULTRY
SOUPS

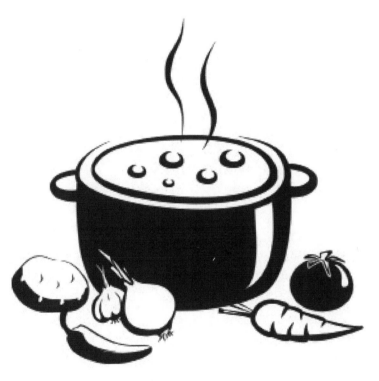

THE
Skinny SLOW
COOKER
SOUP
RECIPE BOOK

Classic Chicken Soup
Serves 4

140 CALORIES PER SERVING

Ingredients:

2 onions, chopped
2 carrots, finely chopped
2 sticks celery, finely chopped
2 garlic cloves, crushed
350g/12oz cooked chicken breast, shredded
1lt/4 cups chicken stock/ broth
Salt & pepper to taste
Low cal cooking oil spray

Method:

• Preheat the slow cooker while you prepare the ingredients.
• Gently sauté the onions, carrots, celery & garlic in a little low cal oil for a few minutes until the onions soften.
• Add all the ingredients to the slow cooker. Combine well, cover and leave to cook on high for 1-1½ hours or until the vegetables are tender.
• Remove 2 ladles of soup and use a blender to blend this to a smooth consistency. Return the blended portion of the soup to the rest of the soup.
• Stir well, season and serve.

Chicken soup is traditionally made with left over shredded chicken. This version uses the leanest cut of the bird - breast meat. Other cuts will have a higher fat content.

Chicken & Mixed Bean Soup

Serves 4

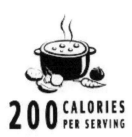

200 CALORIES PER SERVING

Method:

- Preheat the slow cooker while you prepare the ingredients.
- Gently sauté the onion, garlic & celery in a little low cal oil for a few minutes until the onions soften.
- Add all the ingredients to the slow cooker. Combine well, cover and leave to cook on high for 1½-2 hours or until the chicken is cooked through.
- Season and serve.

Ingredients:

1 onion, chopped
2 garlic cloves, crushed
2 celery stalks, chopped
200g/7oz skinless chicken breast, chopped
1 red chilli, deseeded and chopped
1 carrot, chopped
200g/7oz tinned chopped tomatoes
400g/14oz tinned mixed beans, drained
1lt/4 cups chicken stock/ broth
1 tbsp tomato puree/paste
1 tsp dried basil or oregano
Salt & pepper to taste
Low cal cooking oil spray

This is a chunky soup which is should be left unblended. You could add a freshly chopped basil garnish if you like.

Chicken & Fresh Asparagus Soup
Serves 4

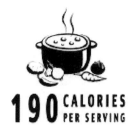

190 CALORIES PER SERVING

Ingredients:

1 onion, chopped
2 garlic cloves, crushed
350g/12oz skinless chicken breast, finely sliced
50g/2oz fine rice noodles
120ml/½ cup dry white wine
1lt/4 cups chicken stock/ broth
200g/7oz fresh asparagus tips, roughly chopped
1 small bunch spring onions/scallions, finely sliced lengthways
Salt & pepper to taste
Low cal cooking oil spray

Method:

• Preheat the slow cooker while you prepare the ingredients.
• Gently sauté the onion & garlic in a little low cal oil for a few minutes until the onions soften.
• Add all the ingredients to the slow cooker, except the asparagus & spring onions. Combine well, cover and leave to cook on high for 1½ hours.
• Add the asparagus and cook for a further 10-20 minutes or until the chicken is cooked through and the asparagus is tender but not overcooked.
• Sprinkle with sliced spring onions, season and serve.

Adding the asparagus towards the end of the cooking time should ensure it still has a little crunch. Feel free to add at the beginning if you prefer it super-tender.

Chicken & Leek Soup

Serves 4

140 CALORIES
PER SERVING

Method:

- Preheat the slow cooker while you prepare the ingredients.
- Gently sauté the onions, garlic & chicken in a little low cal oil for a few minutes until the onions soften.
- Add all the ingredients to the slow cooker. Combine well, cover and leave to cook on high for 1½-2 hours or until the chicken is cooked through and the potatoes are tender.
- Use a blender to blend the soup to your preferred consistency.
- Season and serve.

Ingredients:

1 onion, chopped
2 garlic cloves, crushed
200g/7oz skinless chicken breast, chopped
200g/7oz leeks, sliced
1lt/4 cups chicken stock/ broth
125g/4oz potatoes, chopped
1 tsp dried basil or oregano
Salt & pepper to taste
Low cal cooking oil spray

You could also add some chopped pitted prunes to this soup for a different twist.

Chicken & Sweetcorn Soup
Serves 4

175 CALORIES PER SERVING

Ingredients:

1 onion, chopped
2 garlic cloves, crushed
1 red pepper, sliced
100g/3½oz fresh tomatoes, chopped
200g/7oz skinless chicken breast, chopped
200g/7oz sweetcorn
1lt/4 cups chicken stock/ broth
1 tsp dried basil or coriander/cilantro
Salt & pepper to taste
Low cal cooking oil spray

Method:

• Preheat the slow cooker while you prepare the ingredients.
• Gently sauté the onion, garlic & peppers in a little low cal oil for a few minutes until the onions soften.
• Add all the ingredients to the slow cooker. Combine well, cover and leave to cook on high for 1½-2 hours or until the chicken is cooked through.
• Remove 2 ladles of soup and use a blender to blend this to a smooth consistency. Return the blended portion to the rest of the soup.
• Combine well, season and serve.

Freshly chopped basil or coriander/cilantro makes a lovely garnish to this dish.

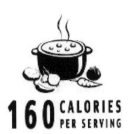

Chicken, Basil & Pepper Soup
Serves 4

160 CALORIES PER SERVING

Method:

- Preheat the slow cooker while you prepare the ingredients.
- Gently sauté the onion, garlic & peppers in a little low cal oil for a few minutes until the onions soften.
- Add all the ingredients to the slow cooker. Combine well, cover and leave to cook on high for 1½-2 hours or until the chicken is cooked through.
- Use a blender to blend the soup to your preferred consistency.
- Check the seasoning and serve.

Ingredients:

1 onion, chopped
2 garlic cloves, crushed
200g/7oz red peppers, sliced
200g/7oz skinless chicken breast, chopped
½ tsp salt
500ml/2 cups chicken stock/broth
500ml/2 cups tomato passata/sieved tomatoes
1 tsp dried basil
Salt & pepper to taste
Low cal cooking oil spray

You could use fresh basil rather than dried if you have it to hand. Save a little for garnishing.

Asian Chicken Soup
Serves 4

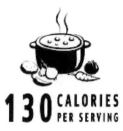

130 CALORIES PER SERVING

Ingredients:

1 onion, chopped
2 garlic cloves, crushed
2 stalks lemongrass, finely chopped
200g/7oz skinless chicken breast, chopped
2 red chillies, finely chopped
2 tbsp soy sauce
1lt/4 cups chicken stock/broth
1 tsp freshly grated ginger
125g/4 oz desiccated coconut
Juice & zest of ½ lime
1 bunch spring onions/scallions, thinly sliced diagonally
Salt & pepper to taste
Low cal cooking oil spray

Method:

• Preheat the slow cooker while you prepare the ingredients.
• Gently sauté the onion, garlic & lemongrass in a little low cal oil for a few minutes until the onions soften.
• Add all the ingredients to the slow cooker, except the spring onions. Combine well, cover and leave to cook on high for 1½-2 hours or until the chicken is cooked through.
• Add the spring onions, check the seasoning and serve.

Freshly chopped coriander/cilantro is a good garnish for this clear Asian soup.

Oriental Chicken & Rice Soup

Serves 4

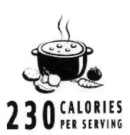

230 CALORIES PER SERVING

Method:

- Preheat the slow cooker while you prepare the ingredients.
- Gently sauté the onion & garlic in a little low cal oil for a few minutes until the onions soften.
- Add all the ingredients to the slow cooker, except the orange juice. Combine well, cover and leave to cook on high for 1½-2 hours or until the chicken is cooked through.
- Remove 2 ladles of soup and use a blender to blend this to a smooth consistency. Return the blended portion to the rest of the soup.
- Add the orange juice, combine well, season and serve.

Ingredients:

1 onion, chopped
2 garlic cloves, crushed
2 carrots, sliced lengthways
200g/7oz skinless chicken breast, chopped
2 tbsp tomato puree/paste
1lt/4 cups chicken stock/ broth
200g/7oz basmati rice
60ml/¼ cup fresh orange juice
1 tsp dried basil or chives
Salt & pepper to taste
Low cal cooking oil spray

Freshly chopped chives make a great garnish for this soup.

Chicken & Pasta Soup
Serves 4

240 CALORIES PER SERVING

Ingredients:

1 onion, chopped
2 garlic cloves, crushed
2 carrots, sliced lengthways
300g/11oz skinless chicken breast, chopped
150g/5oz soup pasta
2 tsp dried mixed herbs
750ml/3 cups chicken stock/broth
Salt & pepper to taste
Low cal cooking oil spray

Method:

• Preheat the slow cooker while you prepare the ingredients.
• Gently sauté the onion & garlic in a little low cal oil for a few minutes until the onions soften.
• Add all the ingredients to the slow cooker. Combine well, cover and leave to cook on high for 1½-2 hours or until the chicken is cooked through and the pasta is tender.
• Season and serve.

Any type of small pasta shape will work for this soup. Add a little grated Parmesan cheese when serving if you wish.

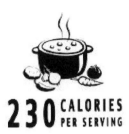

230 CALORIES PER SERVING

Vegetable & Chicken Broth
Serves 4

Method:

- Preheat the slow cooker while you prepare the ingredients.
- Gently sauté the leeks & garlic in a little low cal oil for a few minutes until the leeks soften.
- Add all the ingredients to the slow cooker. Combine well, cover and leave to cook on high for 1½-2 hours or until the chicken is cooked through and the barley is tender.
- Season and serve.

Ingredients:

2 leeks, chopped
2 garlic cloves, crushed
1 carrot, chopped
1 parsnip, chopped
1 turnip, chopped
50g/2oz pre-soaked pearl barley
200g/4oz peas
200g/7oz skinless chicken breast, chopped
2 tsp dried mixed herbs
1lt/4 cups chicken stock/ broth
Salt & pepper to taste
Low cal cooking oil spray

This soup can be blended if you wish or served just as it comes.

Madras Chicken Soup
Serves 4

175 CALORIES PER SERVING

Ingredients:

1 onion, chopped
2 garlic cloves, crushed
2 sticks celery, chopped
1 carrot, chopped
400g/14oz tinned chopped tomatoes
1 tbsp medium curry powder
125g/4oz skinless chicken breast, chopped
100g/3 ½oz basmati rice
500ml/2 cups chicken stock/broth
Salt & pepper to taste
Low cal cooking oil spray

Method:

• Preheat the slow cooker while you prepare the ingredients.
• Gently sauté the onion, garlic & celery in a little low cal oil for a few minutes until the onions soften.
• Add all the ingredients to the slow cooker. Combine well, cover and leave to cook on high for 1½-2 hours or until the chicken is cooked through and the rice is tender.
• Remove 2 ladles of soup and use a blender to blend this to a smooth consistency. Return the blended portion to the rest of the soup.
• Combine well, season and serve.

Freshly chopped coriander/ cilantro adds lovely additional flavour as a garnish for this soup.

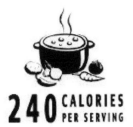

Creamy Chicken & Sweetcorn Soup

Serves 4

240 CALORIES PER SERVING

Method:

- Preheat the slow cooker while you prepare the ingredients.
- Gently sauté the onion in a little low cal oil for a few minutes until softened.
- Add all the ingredients to the slow cooker. Combine well, cover and leave to cook on high for 1½-2 hours or until the chicken is cooked through.
- Discard the bay leaves.
- Remove 2 ladles of soup and use a blender to blend this to a smooth consistency. Return the blended portion to the rest of the soup.
- Combine well, season and serve.

Ingredients:

1 onion, chopped
125g/4oz potatoes, chopped
750ml/3 cups semi skimmed/half fat milk
250ml/1 cup chicken stock/broth
400g/14oz sweetcorn
200g/7oz skinless chicken breast, chopped
½ tsp nutmeg
2 bay leaves
Salt & pepper to taste
Low cal cooking oil spray

You could garnish this soup with freshly chopped chives and a tablespoon of fat free Greek yoghurt.

MEAT SOUPS

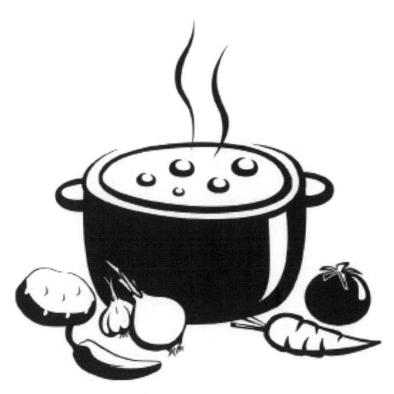

THE
Skinny **SLOW
COOKER
SOUP
RECIPE BOOK**

Beef & Vegetable Broth
Serves 4

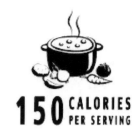

150 CALORIES PER SERVING

Ingredients:

1 leek, chopped
1 onion, chopped
2 garlic cloves, crushed
2 carrots, chopped
50g/2oz pre soaked pearl barley
2 celery sticks, chopped
225g/8oz lean rump steak, finely sliced
1ltml/4 cups beef stock/ broth
Salt & pepper to taste
Low cal cooking oil spray

Method:

• Preheat the slow cooker while you prepare the ingredients.
• Gently sauté the leeks, onion & garlic in a little low cal oil for a few minutes until they soften.
• Add all the ingredients to the slow cooker. Combine well, cover and leave to cook on high for 1½-2 hours or until the vegetables are tender and the steak is cooked through.
• Check the seasoning and serve.

Any cut of beef steak will work fine for this recipe provided it's sliced thinly enough.

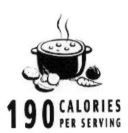

Beef & Bamboo Shoot Soup

Serves 4

190 CALORIES PER SERVING

Method:

• Preheat the slow cooker while you prepare the ingredients.
• Gently sauté the leeks, onion, celery & garlic in a little low cal oil for a few minutes until they soften.
• Add all the ingredients to the slow cooker. Combine well, cover and leave to cook on high for 1½-2 hours or until the vegetables and rice are tender and the steak is cooked through.
• Check the seasoning and serve.

Ingredients:

1 leek, chopped
1 onion, chopped
2 celery sticks, chopped
1 garlic clove, crushed
2 carrots, chopped
1 tbsp soy sauce
2 tbsp tomato puree/paste
75g/3oz long grain rice
125g/4oz tinned bamboo shoots
225g/4oz lean rump steak, finely sliced
1ltml/4 cups beef stock/ broth
Salt & pepper to taste
Low cal cooking oil spray

Chopped fresh chives make a good garnish for this tasty soup.

Spicy Beef Soup
Serves 4

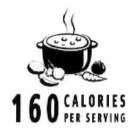

160 CALORIES PER SERVING

Ingredients:

1 onion, chopped
2 garlic cloves, crushed
2 sticks celery, chopped
1 carrot, chopped
400g/14oz tinned chopped tomatoes
2 tbsp tomato puree/paste
1 tbsp medium curry powder
125g/4oz lean rump steak, sliced
100g/3 ½oz basmati rice
500ml/2 cups beef stock/ broth
Salt & pepper to taste
Low cal cooking oil spray

Method:

• Preheat the slow cooker while you prepare the ingredients.
• Gently sauté the onion, garlic & celery in a little low cal oil for a few minutes until the onions soften.
• Add all the ingredients to the slow cooker. Combine well, cover and leave to cook on high for 1½-2 hours or until the beef is cooked through and the rice is tender.
• Remove 2 ladles of soup and use a blender to blend this to a smooth consistency. Return the blended portion to the rest of the soup.
• Combine well, season and serve.

Add some chopped fresh chillies to this soup if you want additional 'heat'.

Pea & Ham Soup

Serves 4

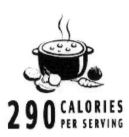

290 CALORIES PER SERVING

Method:

- Preheat the slow cooker while you prepare the ingredients.
- Gently sauté the onion & garlic in a little low cal oil for a few minutes until the onions soften.
- Add all the ingredients to the slow cooker. Combine well, cover and leave to cook on high for 1½-2 hours or until everything is tender.
- Remove 2 ladles of soup and use a blender to blend this to a smooth consistency. Return the blended portion of the soup to the rest of the soup.
- Combine well, season and serve.

Ingredients:

1 onion, chopped
2 garlic cloves, crushed
200g/7oz pre soaked yellow split peas
2 carrots, chopped
2 tsp dried mixed herbs
125g/4oz smoked ham or gammon, chopped
1lt/4 cups chicken stock/ broth
Salt & pepper to taste
Low cal cooking oil spray

Lean ham stripped from a smoked ham hock is ideal for this recipe, but you can use whatever you have to hand.

Oriental Pork Soup
Serves 4

145 CALORIES PER SERVING

Ingredients:

1 onion, chopped
2 garlic cloves, crushed
125g/4oz pork tenderloin, chopped
2 carrots, sliced lengthways
1 bunch spring onions/ scallions sliced lengthways
2 tbsp soy sauce
½ tsp Chinese five spice powder
2 tbsp rice wine vinegar
1 red chilli, finely chopped
200g/7oz tinned water chestnuts
1lt/4 cups chicken stock/ broth
Salt & pepper to taste
Low cal cooking oil spray

Method:

• Preheat the slow cooker while you prepare the ingredients.
• Gently sauté the onion, garlic & pork in a little low cal oil for a few minutes until the onions soften.
• Add all the ingredients to the slow cooker. Combine well, cover and leave to cook on high for 1-1½ hours or until the pork and vegetables are cooked through.
• Season and serve.

Cooked left-over pork is fine to use in this recipe too.

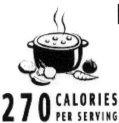

Lentil & Bacon Soup
Serves 4

270 CALORIES PER SERVING

Method:

- Preheat the slow cooker while you prepare the ingredients.
- Gently sauté the onion, garlic & bacon in a little low cal oil for a few minutes until the onions soften.
- Add all the ingredients to the slow cooker. Combine well, cover and leave to cook on high for 1½-2 hours or until everything is tender and cooked through.
- Remove 2 ladles of soup and use a blender to blend this to a smooth consistency. Return the blended portion of the soup to the rest of the soup.
- Combine well, season and serve.

Ingredients:

1 onion, chopped
2 garlic cloves, crushed
125g/4oz lean back bacon, chopped
200g/7oz potatoes, chopped
225g/8oz red lentils
2 carrot, chopped
2 tsp dried mixed herbs
1lt/4 cups chicken stock/ broth
Salt & pepper to taste
Low cal cooking oil spray

Streaky bacon is fine to use too, but it will have a higher fat content.

Beef & New Potato Soup

Serves 4

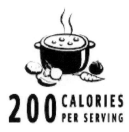

200 CALORIES PER SERVING

Ingredients:

1 leek, chopped
1 onion, chopped
2 garlic cloves, crushed
2 celery sticks, chopped
2 carrots, sliced lengthways
100g/4oz baby sweetcorn cobs, sliced lengthways
200g/7oz baby new potatoes, halved
225g/8oz lean rump steak, finely sliced
1ltml/4 cups beef stock/broth
Salt & pepper to taste
Low cal cooking oil spray

Method:

• Preheat the slow cooker while you prepare the ingredients.
• Gently sauté the leeks, onion, garlic & celery in a little low cal oil for a few minutes until they soften.
• Add all the ingredients to the slow cooker. Combine well, cover and leave to cook on high for 1½-2 hours or until the potatoes and steak are tender and cooked through.
• Check the seasoning and serve.

Any type of halved small or baby potatoes will work well for this recipe, but you could just use chunks of regular potatoes too.

Bacon & Bean Soup

Serves 4

220 CALORIES
PER SERVING

Method:

- Preheat the slow cooker while you prepare the ingredients.
- Gently sauté the leeks, onions, garlic, celery & bacon in a little low cal oil for a few minutes until softened.
- Add all the ingredients to the slow cooker. Combine well, cover and leave to cook on high for 1½-2 hours or until the vegetables and bacon are cooked through.
- Check the seasoning and serve.

Ingredients:

1 leek, chopped
1 onion, sliced
2 garlic cloves, crushed
2 celery stalks, chopped
125g/4oz lean back bacon, chopped
1 carrot, chopped
1 green chilli, finely chopped
400g/14oz tinned mixed beans, drained
2 tbsp tomato puree/paste
1lt/4 cups chicken stock/broth
Salt & pepper to taste
Low cal cooking oil spray

For an alternative twist try using sun-dried tomato puree/paste.

Barley, Lamb & Vegetable Broth
Serves 4

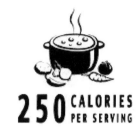

250 CALORIES PER SERVING

Ingredients:

1 leek, chopped
1 onion, chopped
2 garlic cloves, crushed
2 celery sticks, chopped
300g/11oz lean lamb fillet, finely sliced
2 carrots, chopped
50g/2oz pre-soaked pearl barley
1ltml/4 cups beef stock/broth
2 bay leaves
Salt & pepper to taste
Low cal cooking oil spray

Method:

• Preheat the slow cooker while you prepare the ingredients.
• Gently sauté the leeks, onion, garlic, celery & lamb in a little low cal oil for a few minutes until the onions soften.
• Add all the ingredients to the slow cooker. Combine well, cover and leave to cook on high for 1½-2 hours or until the ingredients are cooked through and tender.
• Remove the bay leaves, check the seasoning and serve.

Lamb neck fillet is a good lean choice for this soup.

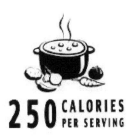

Indian Lamb & Chickpea Soup
Serves 4

250 CALORIES
PER SERVING

Method:

- Preheat the slow cooker while you prepare the ingredients.
- Gently sauté the leeks, onions, garlic & lamb in a little low cal oil for a few minutes softened.
- Add all the ingredients to the slow cooker, except the chopped chilli. Combine well, cover and leave to cook on high for 1½-2 hours or until the ingredients are cooked through and tender.
- Check the seasoning and serve with the chopped chilli sprinkled on top.

Ingredients:

1 leek, chopped
1 onion, chopped
2 garlic cloves, crushed
200g/7oz lean lamb fillet, finely sliced
400g/14oz tinned chopped tomatoes
200g/7oz tinned chickpeas, drained
500ml/2 cups chicken stock/broth
1 tbsp medium curry powder
1 red chilli, finely chopped
Salt & pepper to taste
Low cal cooking oil spray

Freshly chopped coriander/ cilantro makes a great garnish for this soup.

SEAFOOD SOUPS

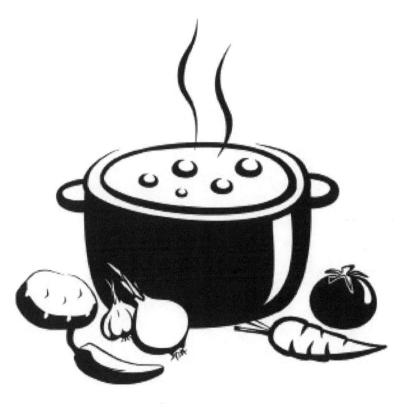

THE
Skinny SLOW
COOKER
SOUP
RECIPE BOOK

Spanish Fish Soup
Serves 4

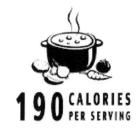

190 CALORIES PER SERVING

Ingredients:

1 onion, chopped
2 garlic cloves, crushed
2 celery stalks, chopped
500g/1lb 2oz skinless
boneless firm fish fillets/
cubed
400g/14oz tinned chopped
tomatoes
500ml/2 cups chicken or
fish stock/broth
1 tsp each dried mixed
herbs & paprika
2 tbsp tomato puree/paste
Salt & pepper to taste
Low cal cooking oil spray

Method:

• Preheat the slow cooker while you prepare the ingredients.
• Gently sauté the onion, garlic & celery in a little low cal oil for a few minutes until the onions soften.
• Add all the ingredients to the slow cooker. Combine well, cover and leave to cook on high for 1-1½ hours or until the fish is cooked through.
• Season and serve.

If you don't have paprika you could add a little chilli instead.

80

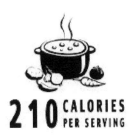

Thai Crab Soup
Serves 4

210 CALORIES PER SERVING

Method:

- Preheat the slow cooker while you prepare the ingredients.
- Add all the ingredients to the slow cooker. Combine well, cover and leave to cook on high for 45mins-1 hour or until the soup is piping hot.
- Season and serve.

Ingredients:

400g/14oz tinned crab meat, drained
2 tbsp Thai red curry paste
750ml/3 cups chicken or fish stock/broth
250ml/1 cup low fat coconut milk
Small bunch spring onions/ scallions, chopped
Salt & pepper to taste
Low cal cooking oil spray

You could use fresh crab meat and/or prawns in this soup along with freshly chopped coriander/cilantro if you have it.

Creamy Crab & Rice Soup
Serves 4

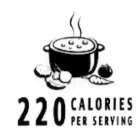

220 CALORIES PER SERVING

Ingredients:

400g/14oz tinned crab meat, drained
100g/3½oz long grain rice
50oml/2 cups chicken or fish stock/broth
500ml/2 cups semi skimmed/half fat milk
1 tsp anchovy paste or 2 tsp Worcestershire sauce
Salt & pepper to taste
Low cal cooking oil spray

Method:

• Preheat the slow cooker while you prepare the ingredients.
• Add all the ingredients to the slow cooker. Combine well, cover and leave to cook on high for 1-1½ hours or until the rice is tender.
• Blend to a smooth consistency, season and serve.

Use anchovy paste if you can as this will give a tasty additional depth to the soup.

82

Smoked Haddock Soup

Serves 4

230 CALORIES PER SERVING

Method:

- Preheat the slow cooker while you prepare the ingredients.
- Add all the ingredients to the slow cooker. Combine well, cover and leave to cook on high for 1-1½ hours or until the potatoes are tender and the fish is cooked through.
- Remove 2 ladles of soup and use a blender to blend this to a smooth consistency. Return the blended portion to the rest of the soup.
- Combine well, season and serve.

Ingredients:

300g/11oz skinless, boneless smoked haddock fillets, cubed
300g/11oz potatoes, peeled & cubed
1lt/4 cups semi skimmed/ half fat milk
1 tsp low fat olive 'butter' spread
Salt & pepper to taste
Low cal cooking oil spray

You could blend all the soup if you prefer a smooth consistency throughout.

Lemongrass Fish Soup
Serves 4

175 CALORIES PER SERVING

Ingredients:

1 onion, chopped
2 garlic cloves, crushed
3 stalks lemongrass, finely chopped
500g/1lb 2oz skinless boneless firm fish fillets/ cubed
3 tbsp Thai fish sauce
1 tsp brown sugar
1 red chilli, finely sliced
1lt/4 cups chicken or fish stock/broth
Salt & pepper to taste
Low cal cooking oil spray

Method:

• Preheat the slow cooker while you prepare the ingredients.
• Gently sauté the onion, garlic & lemongrass in a little low cal oil for a few minutes until the onions soften.
• Add all the ingredients to the slow cooker. Combine well, cover and leave to cook on high for 1-1½ hours or until the fish is cooked through.
• Season and serve.

This soup is great served with lots of freshly chopped coriander/cilantro and lime wedges if you have them.

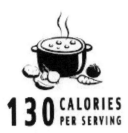

Hot & Sour King Prawn Soup

Serves 4

130 CALORIES PER SERVING

Method:

- Preheat the slow cooker while you prepare the ingredients.
- Gently sauté the onion, garlic & lemongrass in a little low cal oil for a few minutes until the onions soften.
- Add all the ingredients to the slow cooker. Combine well, cover and leave to cook on high for 1-1½ hours or until the prawns are cooked through.
- Season and serve.

Ingredients:

1 onion, chopped
2 garlic cloves, crushed
2 stalks lemongrass, finely chopped
1 tsp freshly grated ginger
400g/14oz shelled king prawns
4 tbsp lime juice
4 tbsp Thai fish sauce
2 red chillies, finely chopped
1 small bunch spring onions/scallions, chopped
125g/4oz mushrooms, sliced
1lt/4 cups chicken or fish stock/broth
Salt & pepper to taste
Low cal cooking oil spray

Kaffir lime leaves make a good garnish but they are not essential.

Prawn & Green Bean Soup
Serves 4

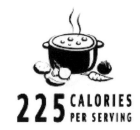

225 CALORIES PER SERVING

Ingredients:

1 onion, chopped
2 garlic cloves, crushed
1 red pepper, sliced
125g/4oz potatoes, chopped
300g/11oz shelled king prawns, roughly chopped
200g/7oz green beans, roughly chopped
200g/7oz tinned chopped tomatoes
750ml/3 cups chicken or fish stock/broth
1 tsp each dried mixed herbs
2 tbsp tomato puree/paste
1 tbsp anchovy paste or 2 tbsp Worcestershire sauce
Salt & pepper to taste
Low cal cooking oil spray

Method:

• Preheat the slow cooker while you prepare the ingredients.
• Gently sauté the onion, garlic & peppers in a little low cal oil for a few minutes until the onions soften.
• Add all the ingredients to the slow cooker. Combine well, cover and leave to cook on high for 1-1½ hours or until the prawns are cooked through and the potatoes are tender.
• Remove 2 ladles of soup and use a blender to blend this to a smooth consistency. Return the blended portion to the rest of the soup.
• Season and serve.

If you don't have anchovy paste or Worcestershire sauce you could add a little cooked streaky bacon for additional salty depth.

86

NOODLE
SOUPS

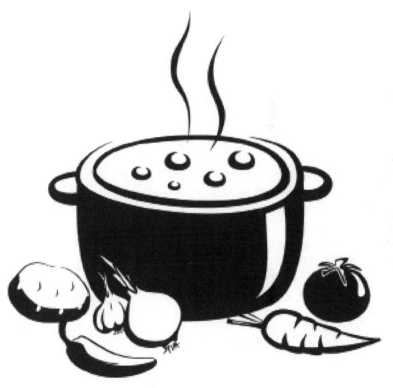

THE

Skinny **SLOW COOKER SOUP RECIPE BOOK**

Pork Noodle Soup
Serves 4

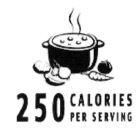

250 CALORIES PER SERVING

Ingredients:

1 onion, chopped
2 garlic cloves, crushed
125g/4oz pork tenderloin,
chopped
2 carrots, sliced
lengthways
1 bunch spring onions/
scallions sliced lengthways
2 tbsp soy sauce
2 tbsp rice wine vinegar
1 tsp freshly grated ginger
1 tsp brown sugar
1 red chilli, finely chopped
200g/7oz tinned bamboo
shoots
1lt/4 cups chicken stock/
broth
150g/5oz fine egg noodles
Salt & pepper to taste
Low cal cooking oil spray

Method:

• Preheat the slow cooker while you
prepare the ingredients.
• Gently sauté the onion, garlic & pork
in a little low cal oil for a few minutes
until the onions soften.
• Add all the ingredients to the slow
cooker. Combine well, cover and leave
to cook on high for 1½-2 hours or until
the pork, vegetables and noodles are
cooked through.
• Season and serve.

*A splash of lime makes a good
garnish for this soup.*

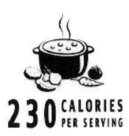

Lemongrass & Noodle Soup

Serves 4

230 CALORIES PER SERVING

Method:

- Preheat the slow cooker while you prepare the ingredients.
- Gently sauté the onion, garlic, lemongrass & pork in a little low cal oil for a few minutes until the onions soften.
- Add all the ingredients to the slow cooker. Combine well, cover and leave to cook on high for 1½-2 hours or until the pork, vegetables and noodles are cooked through.
- Season and serve.

Ingredients:

1 onion, chopped
2 garlic cloves, crushed
2 lemongrass stalks, finely chopped
125g/4oz pork tenderloin, chopped
2 carrots, sliced lengthways
75g/3oz baby sweetcorn, roughly chopped
75g/3oz baby peas
1 bunch spring onions/scallions sliced lengthways
1 red chilli, finely chopped
1lt/4 cups chicken stock/broth
150g/5oz fine egg noodles
Salt & pepper to taste
Low cal cooking oil spray

Add a little freshly chopped flat leaf parsley as a garnish if you have it.

Porcini Noodle Soup
Serves 4

180 CALORIES PER SERVING

Ingredients:

1 onion, chopped
2 garlic cloves, crushed
125g/4oz dried porcini mushrooms, chopped
200g/7oz mushrooms, sliced
1 bunch spring onions/ scallions sliced lengthways
1lt/4 cups vegetable or chicken stock/broth
1 tsp dried rosemary or mixed herbs
150g/5oz fine egg noodles
Salt & pepper to taste
Low cal cooking oil spray

Method:

• Preheat the slow cooker while you prepare the ingredients.
• Gently sauté the onion, garlic & mushrooms in a little low cal oil for a few minutes until softened.
• Add all the ingredients to the slow cooker. Combine well, cover and leave to cook on high for 1-1½ hours or until the mushrooms and noodles are tender and cooked through.
• Season and serve.

Use any type of fresh mushrooms you prefer for this soup.

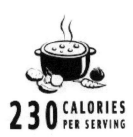

Prawn & Coconut Cream Soup

Serves 4

230 CALORIES PER SERVING

Method:

- Preheat the slow cooker while you prepare the ingredients.
- Gently sauté the onion & garlic in a little low cal oil for a few minutes until softened.
- Add all the ingredients to the slow cooker. Combine well, cover and leave to cook on high for 1-1½ hours or until the prawns and noodles are tender and cooked through.
- Season and serve.

Ingredients:

1 onion, chopped
2 garlic cloves, crushed
125g/4oz sweetcorn
200g/7oz shelled king prawns, roughly chopped
750ml/3 cups vegetable or chicken stock/broth
1 tsp Thai fish sauce
150g/5oz fine egg noodles
2 tbsp coconut cream
Salt & pepper to taste
Low cal cooking oil spray

Finely sliced spring onions make a great garnish for this soup.

Chicken Laksa
Serves 4

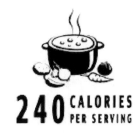

240 CALORIES PER SERVING

Ingredients:

1 onion, chopped
1 leek, sliced
2 garlic cloves, crushed
200g/7oz skinless chicken breast, thinly sliced
2 carrots, sliced lengthways
750ml/3 cups chicken stock/broth
120ml/½ cup low fat coconut milk
150g/5oz thick udon noodles
Salt & pepper to taste
Low cal cooking oil spray

Method:

• Preheat the slow cooker while you prepare the ingredients.
• Gently sauté the onion, leek, garlic & chicken in a little low cal oil for a few minutes until softened.
• Add all the ingredients to the slow cooker. Combine well, cover and leave to cook on high for 1½-2 hours or until the chicken & noodles are tender and cooked through.
• Season and serve.

A pinch of cayenne pepper or chilli powder adds a nice 'kick' to this dish on serving.

Pork & Beansprout Noodle Soup

Serves 4

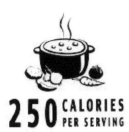

250 CALORIES PER SERVING

Method:

- Preheat the slow cooker while you prepare the ingredients.
- Gently sauté the onion, leek, garlic & pork in a little low cal oil for a few minutes until softened.
- Add all the ingredients to the slow cooker, except the spring onions and beansprouts. Combine well, cover and leave to cook on high for 1½-2 hours or until the pork and noodles are tender & cooked through.
- Add the beansprouts and warm through for a few minutes.
- Serve with the lime wedges.

Ingredients:

1 onion, chopped
1 leek, sliced
2 garlic cloves, crushed
200g/7oz skinless pork tenderloin, finely chopped
1 red chilli, finely chopped
2 carrots, sliced lengthways
75g/3oz sweetcorn
1lt/4 cups chicken stock/broth
150g/5oz medium egg noodles
125g/5oz fresh beansprouts
1 small bunch spring onions/scallions
Lime wedges to serve
Salt & pepper to taste
Low cal cooking oil spray

The beansprouts are added at the end of cooking so that they still have a little crunch. You could add at the beginning of cooking if you prefer.

CONVERSION CHART: DRY INGREDIENTS

Metric	Imperial
7g	¼ oz
15g	½ oz
20g	¾ oz
25g	1 oz
40g	1½oz
50g	2oz
60g	2½oz
75g	3oz
100g	3½oz
125g	4oz
140g	4½oz
150g	5oz
165g	5½oz
175g	6oz
200g	7oz
225g	8oz
250g	9oz
275g	10oz
300g	11oz
350g	12oz
375g	13oz
400g	14oz

Metric	Imperial
425g	15oz
450g	1lb
500g	1lb 2oz
550g	1¼lb
600g	1lb 5oz
650g	1lb 7oz
675g	1½lb
700g	1lb 9oz
750g	1lb 11oz
800g	1¾lb
900g	2lb
1kg	2¼lb
1.1kg	2½lb
1.25kg	2¾lb
1.35kg	3lb
1.5kg	3lb 6oz
1.8kg	4lb
2kg	4½lb
2.25kg	5lb
2.5kg	5½lb
2.75kg	6lb

CONVERSION CHART: LIQUID MEASURES

Metric	Imperial	US
25ml	1fl oz	
60ml	2fl oz	¼ cup
75ml	2½ fl oz	
100ml	3½fl oz	
120ml	4fl oz	½ cup
150ml	5fl oz	
175ml	6fl oz	
200ml	7fl oz	
250ml	8½ fl oz	1 cup
300ml	10½ fl oz	
360ml	12½ fl oz	
400ml	14fl oz	
450ml	15½ fl oz	
600ml	1 pint	
750ml	1¼ pint	3 cups
1 litre	1½ pints	4 cups

Other
COOKNATION
TITLES

If you enjoyed 'The Skinny Slow Cooker Soup Recipe Book' we'd really appreciate your feedback. Reviews help others decide if this is the right book for them so a moment of your time would be appreciated.

Thank you.

You may also be interested in other '**Skinny**' titles in the CookNation series.
You can find all the following great titles by searching under '**CookNation**'.

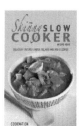

The Skinny Slow Cooker Recipe Book

Delicious Recipes Under 300, 400 And 500 Calories.

Paperback / eBook

More Skinny Slow Cooker Recipes

75 More Delicious Recipes Under 300, 400 & 500 Calories.

Paperback / eBook

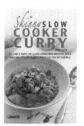

The Skinny Slow Cooker Curry Recipe Book

Low Calorie Curries From Around The World

Paperback / eBook

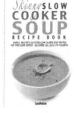

The Skinny Slow Cooker Soup Recipe Book

Simple, Healthy & Delicious Low Calorie Soup Recipes For Your Slow Cooker. All Under 100, 200 & 300 Calories.

Paperback / eBook

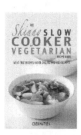

The Skinny Slow Cooker Vegetarian Recipe Book

40 Delicious Recipes Under 200, 300 And 400 Calories.

Paperback / eBook

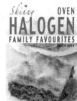

The Skinny 5:2 Slow Cooker Recipe Book

Skinny Slow Cooker Recipe And Menu Ideas Under 100, 200, 300 & 400 Calories For Your 5:2 Diet.

Paperback / eBook

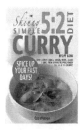

The Skinny 5:2 Curry Recipe Book

Spice Up Your Fast Days With Simple Low Calorie Curries, Snacks, Soups, Salads & Sides Under 200, 300 & 400 Calories

Paperback / eBook

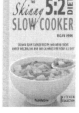

The Skinny Halogen Oven Family Favourites Recipe Book

Healthy, Low Calorie Family Meal-Time Halogen Oven Recipes Under 300, 400 and 500 Calories

Paperback / eBook

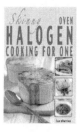

Skinny Halogen Oven Cooking For One

Single Serving, Healthy, Low Calorie Halogen Oven Recipes Under 200, 300 and 400 Calories

Paperback / eBook

Skinny Winter Warmers Recipe Book

Soups, Stews, Casseroles & One Pot Meals Under 300, 400 & 500 Calories.

Paperback / eBook

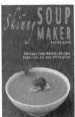

The Skinny Soup Maker Recipe Book

Delicious Low Calorie, Healthy and Simple Soup Recipes Under 100, 200 and 300 Calories. Perfect For Any Diet and Weight Loss Plan.

Paperback / eBook

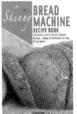

The Skinny Bread Machine Recipe Book

70 Simple, Lower Calorie, Healthy Breads...Baked To Perfection In Your Bread Maker.

Paperback / eBook

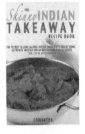

The Skinny Indian Takeaway Recipe Book

Authentic British Indian Restaurant Dishes Under 300, 400 And 500 Calories. The Secret To Low Calorie Indian Takeaway Food At Home

Paperback / eBook

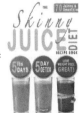

The Skinny Juice Diet Recipe Book

5lbs, 5 Days. The Ultimate Kick-Start Diet and Detox Plan to Lose Weight & Feel Great!

Paperback / eBook

The Skinny 5:2 Diet Recipe Book Collection

All The 5:2 Fast Diet Recipes You'll Ever Need. All Under 100, 200, 300, 400 And 500 Calories

Available only on eBook

eBook

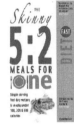

The Skinny 5:2 Fast Diet Meals For One

Single Serving Fast Day Recipes & Snacks Under 100, 200 & 300 Calories

Paperback / eBook

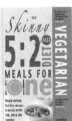

The Skinny 5:2 Fast Diet Vegetarian Meals For One

Single Serving Fast Day Recipes & Snacks Under 100, 200 & 300 Calories

Paperback / eBook

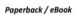
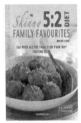

The Skinny 5:2 Fast Diet Family Favourites Recipe Book

Eat With All The Family On Your Diet Fasting Days

Paperback / eBook

The Skinny 5:2 Fast Diet Family Favorites Recipe Book *U.S.A. EDITION*

Dine With All The Family On Your Diet Fasting Days

Available only on eBook

Paperback / eBook

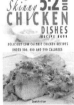

The Skinny 5:2 Diet Chicken Dishes Recipe Book

Delicious Low Calorie Chicken Dishes Under 300, 400 & 500 Calories

Paperback / eBook

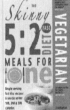

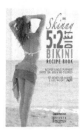

The Skinny 5:2 Bikini Diet Recipe Book

Recipes & Meal Planners Under 100, 200 & 300 Calories. Get Ready For Summer & Lose Weight...FAST!

Paperback / eBook

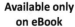

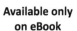

The Paleo Diet For Beginners Slow Cooker Recipe Book

Gluten Free, Everyday Essential Slow Cooker Paleo Recipes For Beginners

Available only on eBook

eBook

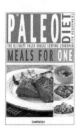

The Paleo Diet For Beginners Meals For One

The Ultimate Paleo Single Serving Cookbook

Paperback / eBook

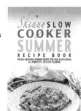

The Paleo Diet For Beginners Holidays

Thanksgiving, Christmas & New Year Paleo Friendly Recipes

Available only on eBook

eBook

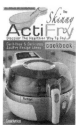
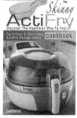

The Healthy Kids Smoothie Book

40 Delicious Goodness In A Glass Recipes for Happy Kids.

eBook

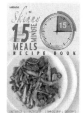

The Skinny Slow Cooker Summer Recipe Book

Fresh & Seasonal Summer Recipes For Your Slow Cooker. All Under 300, 400 And 500 Calories.

Paperback / eBook

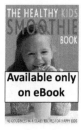

The Skinny ActiFry Cookbook

Guilt-free and Delicious ActiFry Recipe Ideas: Discover The Healthier Way to Fry!

Paperback / eBook

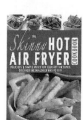

The Skinny 15 Minute Meals Recipe Book

Delicious, Nutritious & Super-Fast Meals in 15 Minutes Or Less. All Under 300, 400 & 500 Calories.

Paperback / eBook

The Skinny Mediterranean Recipe Book

Simple, Healthy & Delicious Low Calorie Mediterranean Diet Dishes. All Under 200, 300 & 400 Calories.

Paperback / eBook

The Skinny Hot Air Fryer Cookbook

Delicious & Simple Meals For Your Hot Air Fryer: Discover The Healthier Way To Fry.

Paperback / eBook

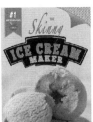
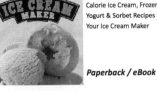

The Skinny Ice Cream Maker

Delicious Lower Fat, Lower Calorie Ice Cream, Frozen Yogurt & Sorbet Recipes For Your Ice Cream Maker

Paperback / eBook

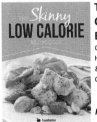

The Skinny Low Calorie Recipe Book

Great Tasting, Simple & Healthy Meals Under 300, 400 & 500 Calories. Perfect For Any Calorie Controlled Diet.

Paperback / eBook

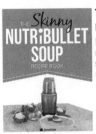

The Skinny Takeaway Recipe Book

Healthier Versions Of Your Fast Food Favourites: Chinese, Indian, Pizza, Burgers, Southern Style Chicken, Mexican & More. All Under 300, 400 & 500 Calories

Paperback / eBook

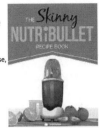

The Skinny Nutribullet Recipe Book

80+ Delicious & Nutritious Healthy Smoothie Recipes. Burn Fat, Lose Weight and Feel Great!

Paperback / eBook

The Skinny Nutribullet Soup Recipe Book

Delicious, Quick & Easy, Single Serving Soups & Pasta Sauces For Your Nutribullet. All Under 100, 200, 300 & 400 Calories.

Paperback / eBook

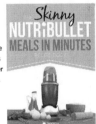

The Skinny Nutribullet Meals In Minutes Recipe Book

Quick & Easy, Single Serving Suppers, Snacks, Sauces, Salad Dressings & More. All Under 300, 400 & 500 Calories.

Paperback / eBook

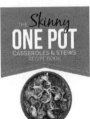

The Skinny One-Pot Recipe book

Simple & Delicious, One-Pot Meals. All Under 300, 400 & 500 Calories

Paperback / eBook

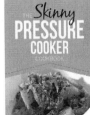

The Skinny Pressure Cooker Cookbook

"USA ONLY"

Low Calorie, Healthy & Delicious Meals, Sides & Desserts. All Under 300, 400 & 500 Calories.

Paperback / eBook

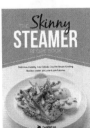

The Skinny Steamer Recipe Book

Delicious, Healthy, Low Calorie, Low Fat Steam Cooking Recipes Under 300, 400 & 500 Calories

Paperback / eBook

Printed in Great Britain
by Amazon.co.uk, Ltd.,
Marston Gate.